"How to be Healthy and Heal the Body with Recipes for Life!!"

By Dr. John Bergman

Disclaimer

You must not rely on the information in this book and/or video series as an alternative to medical advice from your doctor or other professional healthcare provider. If you have any specific questions about any medical matter, you should consult your doctor or other professional healthcare provider.

If you think you may be suffering from any medical condition, you should seek immediate medical attention. You should never delay seeking medical advice, disregard medical advice, or discontinue medical treatment because of information in this book and/or video series.

Any change in medication, diet, and/or exercise should be directed by a qualified health care professional.

This book is dedicated to my mom

I was born in 1960. I was the youngest of 4 children and the only boy. I am so lucky to have had such an amazing family. My 3 sisters were supportive and full of love. Since my mom worked so much my sisters raised me and I learned a lot from them and I still do. When I was 4 years old my parents got divorced, so I found out what it was like to be raised by a single working mom with 3 teenage sisters in the turbulent 1960's. When my parents were divorced it devastated my father and he wasn't able to help financially or emotionally. It took him years to become involved in our family and my memory of him is of a kind loving man who cared deeply. He died when I was 14 years old, so I didn't have him for long, but the time I had with him affected my life deeply. He taught me honor, respect and love.

My Mom worked for the movie and TV studios in Burbank and Hollywood, California.

She worked in casting and move up from a secretary to an assistant casting director. She had the ability to be successful at work and still maintain a loving strong safe home. My mom taught me how to cook before I was old enough to know how to cook. Sunday night my mom would make a huge dinner and would save the leftovers for Monday night, storing them in containers in the refrigerator with aluminum foil on top.

I was a true "latch key kid". In the first grade our house key hung on a piece of white yarn around my neck so when I got home from school I could let myself in. First thing I did when I got home was sit in front of the TV and watch cartoons. When I went to the fridge for a snack there would be a note on the fridge, "Preheat the oven to 350 degrees at 5 pm". There would be a note on the food containers "place them in the oven one at 5:15pm, the other containers at 5:30pm".When my sisters and mom got home at 6pm our home would smelled great! My sisters made such a big deal about "who made the dinner?" Mom would always say, "John made it". The way my mom arranged meals was: Sunday big meal, Monday leftovers, Tuesday she would add pasta or potatoes to extend the meal, Wednesday leftovers and by Thursday it would be soup and Friday was "live it up night" and we would go out to some type of fast food or restaurant.

The foods that we ate in the 1960's were radically different from the foods we eat today. There were no Genetically Modified foods, No Growth hormones, few antibiotics were used in the animals we ate. Today, we must modify how and what we eat. Most of my mom's recipes would not work today. Mom made us a breakfast of: orange juice and gelatin and any other fruits she had for a "power drink" to start the day. This was very advanced for the 1960's. At that time there were no health food stores and mom would have been considered a "health nut". She passed a few years ago, but she is still with me in my heart. I love her still.

In all my health talks I say "I was raise with strong powerful women" now my readers also know.

Table of Contents

Chapter 1:

A Guide to Health

This book of recipes is for optimal healing. Your body is self-healing, self-regenerating and self-regulating. Nutrition isn't taught in detail in Medical schools, even though throughout time even the "father of medicine" Hippocrates said "Let food be your medicine and medicine be your food." Older than that there is an Ayurvedic saying "when diet is good medicine is of no need and when diet is poor medicine is of no good." This book is to guide you on how your body metabolizes nutrients, prevent and even reverse disease in most cases.

I will present information so my readers can get the most out of the food they eat where ever they live on our planet. Certain areas won't have fresh vegetables available year round, so I will ask you to substitute fermented vegetables and show you how to prepare them.

You may not have access to fresh coconuts or fresh spices. I will always give you alternatives so no matter where you are or what you can afford you will always have cost effective healthy food choices for you and your family. I will also show you how to have healthy meals that even the pickiest child or adult will like.

Diseases start in the gut, so we have to heal the gut first. You will need some equipment to predigest your food. Most people today have poor digestion from the types of food available and poor medical care. They overuse medications and have poor quality of foods.

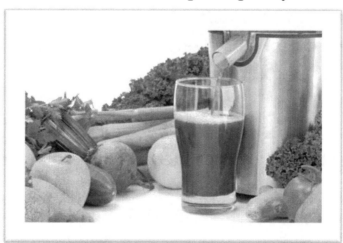

You will need a juicer and a blender. The difference is a juicer will separate heavy fibers from soluble fibers. A blender breaks down the whole fruits or vegetables at high speed and keeps the whole foods together. The best juicer will be a slow speed masticating. I recommend the Omega VRT-350®.I have used the Champion®, Brevile®, and Green Star®, they all have advantages and disadvantages. Find the juicer that works best for you. The faster speed juicers will oxidize the juice which makes it not last as long and may destroy some vital enzymes.

The best blender that I have found is the Blendtec®. The Vitamix® is also an excellent blender. If you can't afford a new juicer or blender look for a used one, you can also find great deals at garage sales.

Sweeteners:

Use a natural sweetener such as honey, organic cane sugar, pure maple syrup grade B, or coconut sugar. Do Not use synthetic sweeteners as <u>Aspartame or Saccharine</u>. If you have diabetes try <u>Stevia</u> liquid for sweetener.

Cooking:

Do not use a microwave.

Use an <u>electric toaster oven</u> for fast heating, or a gas, electric, or alcohol stove.

Do Not Use Plastic Wrap:

The chemicals in plastic wrap can leach into contents of foods and beverages.

For cooking temperature try to make sure you keep most foods heated to 118 degrees or lower to maintain the enzyme integrity with at least 80% of your meals.

Cookware:

Use no aluminum (pots or rice cookers). Preferred is glass, ceramic coated steel (find good used ones at estate sales) or heavy stainless steel. Use <u>no aluminum foil</u> for food storage or cooking. Use <u>no Styrofoam</u> or <u>soft plastic</u> for storage of water, beverages or food. Avoid non-stick tephlon® cook ware, or aluminum pots and pans they can be toxic.

Healthy Oils

Make sure you avoid all polyunsaturated oils. No Corn oil, No Soy oil, No Canola oil, etc… Most oils become rancid quickly at room temperature. Some oils are great, like flax oil for reversing some diseases but they must be made fresh from ground flax seeds to be effective. The best oils to use are the saturated oils like: Coconut oil, Palm oil, Ghee butter, and Organic Butter from healthy goats or cows. Make sure you avoid commercially produced animal fats, they are toxic and dangerous. Organic olive oil is great, just try to use it with low heat or raw.

Grains

The best grains to use are ancient grains like quinoa, buckwheat, organic wild rice, etc.For any other grains you use make sure they are sprouted and organic. You want to avoid any commercially produced gains like most wheat and soy products. The wheat I grew up with compared to today's wheat is completely different. What used to be healthy may now be toxic.

Animal Products

Avoid any commercially produced animal products. The way we raise animals at our factory farms is sick and cruel for both the animals and the consumer. I encourage you to read "Diet for the new America" by John Robbins. When I read that book it changed my view of our relationship to our planet and our connection to all the species here on earth. I know going vegan may not be possible for many people, so try to consume humanly raised animals and make sure it is a small part of your calorie intake.

Canned and Packaged Foods

Canned and packaged foods are sometimes preserved with toxic chemicals. Most canned foods used to be safe, now most cans are lined with a type of plastic called BPA. BPA can cause cancer and weaken your immune system. Even organic vegetables canned in BPA lined cans can be toxic. The next chapter on fermented foods will teach you how to prepare your own healthy vegetables and have them all year. Also, avoid foods such as; processed foods with additives, soy foods (unless traditionally fermented), and refined sugar. There are many alternatives to refined sugar, for example; raw sugar, coconut crystals, honey, agave, and Stevia.

Many health conditions that people are suffering from like: Autism, Attention Deficit Disorder, Anxiety, Bipolar Disorder, Depression, Irritable Bowel Syndrome, Crohn's Disease, and many other diseases begin in the gut. To heal the gut it's vital to go **Gluten free** and **Casein free**.

Gluten is the protein found in wheat, rye, barley, commercial oats (there are gluten free oats available), kamut and spelt. There are many products today that are made gluten-free.

Casein is the protein found in dairy, processed cow milk, cheese, yogurt, etc. There are many alternatives that can be substituted for dairy, such as, almond milk, and coconut milk.

Chapter 2: Fermentation

I have a video on how to ferment foods:

http://www.youtube.com/watch?v=TiigsFnND
uQ

The fermentation of vegetables and meats has been used for centuries before refrigeration was available. Without fermentation we wouldn't have cheese, beer, wine, or sauerkraut. Fermentation allows healthy bacteria to be introduced into your system. Without healthy bacteria you wouldn't be able to digest most of your food. Healthy bacteria protects you from dangerous bacteria and viruses. A healthy body has about 70 trillion cells and about 4 times that number of bacteria. With the standard medical overuse of antibiotics and the massive use of antibiotics in commercial farm animals, this has caused a huge deficit of healthy bacteria in most people.

Have fun with fermentation! Start with cabbage, then branch out to carrots, beets, salsa, peppers, coconut water, add in onions, garlic, jalapeno's, and anything you can think of. The basic process of fermentation is to cut the vegetables as small as possible to increase surface area and allow the fermentation process to occur. The first step is to get wide mouth quart glass jars, healthy sea salt and spring water or purified water.

Start with any fresh, washed vegetable that you'd like. Cut into small pieces and use sea salt liberally to bring the water out of the veggies. Mix veggies and salt in a large bowl, squeezing and mixing the veggies at the same time. Next, pack your veggie mixture in the jars making sure you pack it down to get all of the air out. Air is the only thing that can cause mold to form during the fermentation process. That is the main thing you want to avoid.

Pack the veggies in the jars to get the air out. You will see water start to come to the surface. You need to make sure that there is little to no air in the jar. Let the jars of newly packed veggies sit out on your counter, away from direct sunlight, at room temperature, for 7 to 10 days. There will be pressure that builds up during the fermenting process and some leakage will occur through the tops of your fermenting jars. Make sure you place the jars on a cookie sheet or pan to catch the fluid. Try the veggies after a few days to test the flavor. You may want to stop the fermentation early or let it go for some more time. Once your veggies are where you want them to be, stop the fermentation process. You do this by simply putting them into the refrigerator. A great book on fermentation is "The art of fermentation" By: Sandor Katz.

The introduction of fermented foods is vital for healing a gut in a person with Fibromyalgia, Depression, Anxiety, Attention Deficit Disorder, Reflux, Irritable Bowel Syndrome, and many more dis-eases. If you don't use or like fermented foods then you may need to take probiotics to repair your gut bacteria called "normal flora". Probiotics are living bacteria that allow your natural intestinal bacteria to grow to healthy levels. I can't stress enough how important healthy gut bacteria is for healthy digestion and disease reversal.

Heating your fermented foods above 118 degrees can kill the healthy bacteria that you need, so make sure you lightly sauté or eat your delicious fermented foods raw. This is also a great way to have fresh veggies year round no matter where you live. Fermented foods have been a staple of mankind for centuries. It is time to reintroduce them back into our culture and regain our health.

Chapter 3:

The Physiology of Food and How to Clean the Arteries

Foods can open up blood vessels, lower or raise blood pressure, change your moods, increase or decrease your immune system. The foods you chose to put into your body will effect what you need to regain your health or cause disease. Let's start by looking at blood vessels. In your body you have arteries and veins. Arteries have three layers, an inner lining called endothelium, a muscular layer, and an outer layer. Arteries can open or dilate or constrict as needed. There are also vasa vasorums, or the blood vessels of the blood vessels. Arteries have their own blood supply. Many diseases start with consuming foods that damage the endothelium or the inner lining of the arteries. Animal products can cause this inner lining to inflame and slow down the natural blood flow.

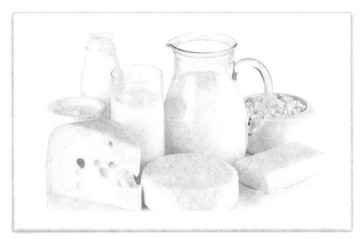

Dairy

Dairy has many benefits; however, if the dairy is homogenized and pasteurized this processing turns a healthy product into something that can damage the endothelium. In the old days when a milk man brought dairy products to the home, the dairy was unprocessed and from healthy animals. Milk would separate; the cream would float to the top of the milk jars. The quality of the milk was measured by how much cream was in the jars. The processing of dairy called **Homogenization** is done by blasting the raw milk with thousands of pounds of pressure into a steel plate breaking the healthy large milk fats into shards of fat diffusing out the fat into the milk. This process allowed the dairy industry to get away with less cream in the milk so it was a cheaper milk product. In turn, the dairy industry was able to profit by keeping more cream for butter and cheese. The problem with the homogenization process is that the shards of fats created can damage and inflame the artery lining.

The **pasteurization** process allows for a longer shelf life of the dairy products. Pasteurization was first brought on to kill dangerous bacteria that can be found in milk, if the milk is obtained from unhealthy animals or from unhealthy conditions. Milk is produced from cows, sheep, goats and humans only when they are nursing babies after they have given birth. Most commercial dairies use hormones to keep cows continually producing milk in extremely unhealthy conditions. A real dairy cow can live 20 years, a commercial dairy cow is lucky to live 5 years. Unhealthy animals will give you an unhealthy product.

Raw dairy can help reverse many diseases, homogenized and pasteurized dairy can be dangerous and can promote disease. In the U.S.A. we have a government agency called the F.D.A. or the Food and Drug Administration. The FDA is mainly concerned with the health of industrial food production and corporate interests instead of the health of the consumers of the food products. It is up to the consumer to read labels and demand healthy foods and food processing. The sad state of the commercial dairy industry in regards to the quality of the products and the health of the animals is just one example of the failure of the F.D.A. Organic dairies need to be supported from the grass roots level. Ethical treatment of the animals is vital if we want a healthy planet, and a healthy population.

Commercially produced chickens, pork, beef, and lamb are also toxic to your arteries. 70% of all the antibiotics used in this country are used in commercial animal feeds. This use of antibiotics allows the animals to be kept alive long enough to get fat enough to slaughter. These government approved commercial farming practices are a major cause of the chronic diseases that most Americans suffer from today. When I say your food **must** be organic it is mandatory to obtain health. Consuming animal products from these factory farms can damage the lining of the arteries.

Now let's look at how to clean the arteries. There are 2 types of fibers in plants soluble and insoluble fibers. Soluble fibers are fibers that can clean arteries. Insoluble fibers can help clean the colon. Juicing is the best way to obtain the soluble fibers. The difference between juicing and blending is that a juicer separates the heavy fibers (insoluble fibers) from the small fibers (soluble fibers). The advantage of a blender is that you can blend whole fruit or vegetable getting both the soluble and insoluble fibers. Blenders are great for fruits, because you can use the whole fruit to get the all the benefits. The disadvantage of blenders is that the high speed tends to oxidize the juice and may destroy some enzymes. Also, it doesn't separate the insoluble fibers from the soluble fibers. This process of getting the soluble fibers separated is vital for cleaning the arteries. Heavy fibers (insoluble) are great for cleaning the intestinal track and very necessary for health. I recommend the following tasty and nutritious juice formula that produces about 10, 32-oz mason jars of juice.

Three 3lb bags of apples,
Two 5 lb bags of carrots
Six bundles of spinach
Three bundles of celery

Special add-ons for juice:
Garlic for colds/flues
Ginger for stomach issues
Kale for strong immune system and iron

Bell peppers for extra vit. C
Organic Strawberries
Beets + Beet Greens

Put the juice in mason jars and over-fill them so when you put the top on there are no air pockets. Refrigerate the juice right away. The juice should stay fresh from 24 to 72 hours, depending on the juicer. High speed juicers will introduce a lot of oxygen and degrade the juice faster. A slow speed, masticating juicer will make the juice stay fresh longer.
Get creative with juicing and use a variety of vegetables. When you prepare broccoli for cooking, save the stalks for juicing later, in fact, most veggie parts that you would normally throw away are good for your juice. I like the formula above because the apples have malic acid, which is great for cleaning arteries (leave the core in the apple when you juice). Spinach is loaded with protein, carrots help with lung function (for detoxing), and celery is

great for minerals. Add anything you want: kale, fennel, any dark green veggies.
Blending is great for fruits. You need to blend fruits, not juice them, but apples are an exception. Apples can be both blended and juiced. Blending is awesome for a fast breakfast or a quick meal. My favorite blending formulas are:

Coconut Smoothie: a good post workout or breakfast.
1 young Thai coconut, 1 frozen banana, 1 scoop veggie raw protein powder, 2 Tbsp raw cacao chips or powder, 1 scoop spirulina.

Papaya, mango, banana, smoothie: Great for parasites and to heal the gut.
Peel 1 papaya but make sure put the papaya and the seed in the blender, add 1 frozen banana, the fruit of a medium mango, 2 cups of spring water, 1 scoop of spirulina, a handful of ice. Blend and enjoy.

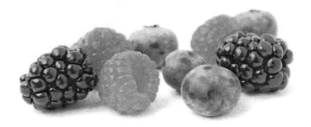

Berry smoothie a great breakfast or desert: 2 handfuls of organic fresh or frozen berries (blue berries, raspberries, black berries, etc…), 1 frozen banana, a scoop of raw cacao, 2 cups of spring water or a handful of ice. Blend and enjoy

The health of the arteries is the first step in regaining health and reversing disease. To break this down to simple terms, don't eat things that will inflame the artery linings. Eat foods that will heal and clean the arteries.

Chapter 4:

Genetically Modified Foods

In the U.S.A. today, we have a population that is both obese and starving at the same time. This is a population that is starving for healthy nutrients. Anytime you see someone who is obese, what they're doing is taking in nutrients that they're *not* digesting. So the body naturally stores the nutrients.

Since the standard American diet is loaded with toxic fats, Genetically Modified Organisms (GMOs), preservatives, and chemical flavorings, this means that the population is toxic. We have to deal these toxins if we are going to correct High Blood Pressure. There are a number of steps:

First we have to eliminate GMOs. There are no human studies, but there are a few animal studies that show identified health risks associated with GM food consumption:

- Infertility

- Immune system compromise
- Accelerated aging

Altered genes associated with:

- cholesterol synthesis
- insulin regulation
- cell signaling
- protein formation

Alterations in function of:

- liver
- kidney
- spleen
- gut function

Many countries in the world do not allow GMO crops because of the known health risks and the unknown consequences when it comes to human consumption.

In the U.S.A. the approved GMOs, including those foods that have been genetically "modified" include:

- Herbicide resistance
- Corn, soy, cotton, canola, rice, alfalfa, beet, flax

- Insect resistance (Pesticide Prod)
- Corn, cotton, potato, tomato
- Sterile pollen (Terminator Tech)
- Corn, chicory
- Virus resistance
- Papaya, squash,
- Plum
- Delayed ripening Tomato
- Altered oil
- Canola, soy
- Protein composition
- Corn
- Reduced nicotine tobacco

The only way to be safe and to not consume toxic food is to get 100% organic food. Some people will say that organic food is too "expensive". There are many ways to buy organic at a discount: buy direct from farmers markets, talk directly to the farmer to find out if the food is grown without pesticides, use all of the plants (use the beat greens, use the broccoli stems and leaves, make soups out of the heavy fibers from your juicing, etc..). What you eat becomes YOU, so choose quality. The recipes that I have at the end of this book are both economical and delicious. Follow them to reverse disease and obtain optimal health.

Chapter 5:

Clear, Clean, Water, and Healthy Fats

It's very important to be fully hydrated. This means you need to drink healthy water at the rate of about 50% of your body weight in ounces every day. That means a 200 lb person needs 100 ounces of water every day. As vital as water is, make sure you drink **no** water ½ hour before, ½ hour after meals and drink little to no water during meals. The reason for this restriction is that water can dilute the stomach acids that you need to digest your food. Too much water with meals is a major cause of indigestion and reflux.

Water is a good blood thinner, a great pain reliever, a fantastic method of detoxing, and the most vital nutrient you need. The main problem with the water most people are exposed to is the toxins in it. Water today is fluoridated, chlorinated, or packaged in toxic containers. Filtering today's water is vital to your survival. Water packaged in plastic containers is not regulated by the FDA unless it crosses state lines. I encourage everyone to watch the movie **Tapped** to understand what is happening with the bottled water industry. First you need a filter that filters out the fluoride, eliminates chloride, chlorine, heavy metals, bacteria, and drugs. Healthy water is the key to healthy metabolic function.

The most cost effective water filter that I have found is from www.doultonusa.com. I use the counter top model. It removes fluoride and most of the toxins that are in our water supply. Become proactive with your communities water source. Vote down any fluoridation of your water system. The majority of people I see are not getting close to the healthy amount of water they need daily. With the right water intake, there is a huge number of diagnoses or diseases that could be cured with simply the right water intake. I encourage you to read

"Your Body's Many Cries for Water" by Dr. Batamanghelidj. It is a brilliant and well-researched book on diseases that can be cured by sufficient water intake.

Below is a talk I gave on the importance of healthy water….

https://www.youtube.com/watch?v=nb6ttXxb5 tU

Healthy fats vs. unhealthy fats. First let's start with fats you need to avoid. Eliminate Poly Unsaturated Fatty Acids, also called PUFAs. PUFAs are in almost all packaged foods, and they are canola oil, soy oil, safflower oil, and most seed oils. PUFAs cause blood vessels to clump together. Blood vessels are shaped like a bi-concaved disc, like two Frisbees® glued together. This design holds the maximum amount of oxygen. If the blood vessels are clumped together, they can't hold a good amount of oxygen and the blood gets thicker, so pressure has to increase to get that unhealthy blood through the arteries. PUFA's also inflame the lining of your arteries called systemic inflammation. Systemic inflammation acidifies your body leading to diseases like Cancer, Dementia, Arthritis, High Blood Pressure. Over 90% of diseases have their origins in an acidic body.

Healthy oils are organic cold pressed olive oil, organic raw coconut oil and organic palm oil.

Make sure if you use olive oil you heat it to no more than 118 degrees to maintain its healthy properties. Healthy fats are vital for a healthy thyroid and adrenal function. Both of these are needed for a healthy body, disease resistance and reversal. I recommend on average about 3 Tbsp. of coconut oil per day for the average person. Follow your doctor's recommendation for oils. Some people may have medical conditions that will cause difficulty to digest oils. Keep in mind though that most doctors have no training in nutrition, so make sure your doctor has experience and is educated on the effects of diet and its effect on the disease process.

Coconut oil doesn't require a gall bladder for absorption, whereas other oils do. If you have had your gall bladder removed, this may be a good option for you. Coconut oil is a medium chain fatty acid and it is excellent for restoring brain function. A healthy brain burns glucose, but if you have leaky gut syndrome (which most people have, due to antibiotics, vaccinations, and exposure to pesticides in commercially produced foods) large proteins, usually from gluten (from grains) and caseins (from dairy), can attach to opiate receptors (pleasure sensors) in the brain. This action of blocking the receptor sites is very common in patients with High Blood Pressure, Attention Deficit Disorder (ADD), Autism Spectrum Disorders (ASD) and Fibromyalgia Syndrome (FMS). This causes an almost starving of the brain. It is essential to go on a gluten-free, dairy-free diet and get at least 1to 5 Tbsp. of raw organic coconut oil daily to heal the brain. Most oils become rancid at room temperature however the tropical oils like coconut and palm oil stay fresh at room temperature.

Chapter 6:

Stress and Digestion

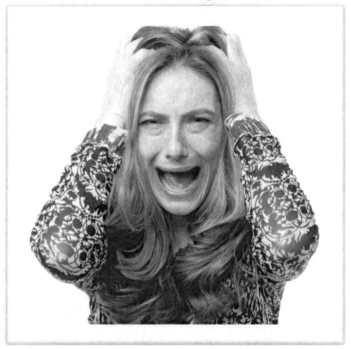

Stress can be broken down to 3 different types: Physical, Chemical, and Emotional. The body's response to physical, chemical and emotional stress is basically all *the same*. What this means is how your body responses to an auto accident, from a *neurologic* perspective, is the same as if you were under Chemical stress (toxic food, medications, environmental toxins) or Emotional stress. Under physical, chemical or emotional stress, your body activates the fight-or-flight system or Sympathetic Nervous System (SNS). The SNS is what all species on this planet have and use to keep alive in the short term and it is a natural response to danger. When this SNS kicks into active mode, blood supply to the gut is shut down, heart rate is elevated, immune system is weakened, blood sugar is elevated, and cholesterol is elevated. All the types of stress cause a sympathetic dominant pattern. For healthy digestion you need to break out of this sympathetic dominant pattern and restore normal nervous system function so the body can go back to its *normal state of Health*. To recover healthy digestion, you have to get your nervous system functioning correctly.

To understand this fight or flight response, we have to look at the other half of the autonomic nervous system, or the "Rest, Digest and

Repair system," also called the Parasympathetic Nervous System (PNS). You have an *automatic* nervous system called the "autonomic nervous system." This does all of those functions that are vital for life but are way too complicated to do consciously. When you're at rest, your heart slows down, when you're active your heart and kidney functions increase. Your body digests food with saliva from your mouth. To digest carbohydrates, stomach acids are produced to digest proteins and bile from your liver is secreted to digest fats. All this goes on without you consciously knowing or thinking about it. If you cut yourself, histamines are released and millions of cells go to work to regenerate new skin and repair blood vessels. In fact, your entire body is replaced at an amazing rate.

- Bones are replaced every 8 to 11 months

- The lining in the stomach and intestine, every 4 days

- The gums are replaced every 2 weeks

- The skin is replaced every 4 weeks
- The liver is replaced every 6 weeks
- The lining of blood vessels is replaced every 6 months

This constant renewability of your body is a fact what is missed and unappreciated by most doctors and most of the public today. The purpose of every book I write, and every lecture I have given over the last 16 years is to change people's perception and emphasize the true beauty and amazing nature of our human body. This constant repair and rebuilding process must occur or our systems would break down. The body is never static, it's either breaking down or rebuilding. For individuals that are in a chronic fight or flight state, the body breaks down faster than it is able to regenerate. Since *that* is the source of most diseases, then the solution of disease will be in dealing with and correcting the stressors.

Correcting physical stress may require reversal of arthritis or regeneration of the structures of the body like the spinal discs. You may need to change your work environment or some of the physical stress you have on a day to day basis. I recommend that you get your nervous system checked for physical stress by a corrective Chiropractor first.

Correcting Chemical stress requires you to take in healthy nutrients and check any medications you have been prescribed. Typically medications are given to alter your physiology like blood pressure, cholesterol, blood sugar, depression, etc.. All those symptoms are eliminated usually when you correct the stressors that caused that response. Most of the medications that are prescribed are given to alter a stressed physiology and do nothing to correct the cause of the stress. Correcting emotional stress requires you to change your perception. There are several techniques that need to be learned for good emotional health.

Below is a health talk I gave demonstrating some of those techniques:

http://www.youtube.com/watch?v=He_uTsFS mYY

Chapter 7

Kitchen Basic Herbs, Spices, and Veggies

"Let food be your medicine and medicine be your food" -Hippocrates
Herbs and spices have been used for centuries for their healing properties. I'm going to cover the basic ones that are essential have in your kitchen.

Cayenne pepper = *Vasodilator*- It will open blood vessels and help your heart and kidney function. It comes in pill form and needs to be taken immediately before meals or it will upset your stomach.

Sea salt=make sure it is dark brown, gray or pink in color. This means it has a good amount of minerals. Sea salt will lower blood pressure and help with joint pain. You need healthy minerals for every cellular function of your body.

Black pepper= helps with digestion and tastes good.

Turmeric= has fantastic healing properties including anti-tumor effects and its active ingredient are Curcumin.

Curcumin= Awesome healing properties and taste great. Curcumin has been a potential treatment for an array of diseases, including Cancer, Alzheimer's, diabetes, allergies, arthritis and other chronic illnesses.

Garlic = great anti-microbial. Garlic was used to kill bad bacteria and viruses for centuries. In WWI they used garlic paste to prevent wound infections.

Onions= great for the immune system and can clean your blood. Contains Anti-Inflammatory, and Anti-cholesterol properties.

Chile's Jalapeño = Great for opening blood vessels and loaded with vitamin C.

Oregano = has anti-microbial properties great for your immune system.

Basil = Great for your immune system

Cinnamon= Great for your immune system, and balancing blood sugar levels.

Hemp seeds = loaded with omega-3's

Chia seeds= loaded with omega-3's

Raw Cacao powder = Great source of minerals. This is chocolate in its raw form without the sugar or fat.

Maca root powder = great for immune system and hormone production and hormone balance.

Nutmeg = aids in Adrenal support.

Vital vegetables

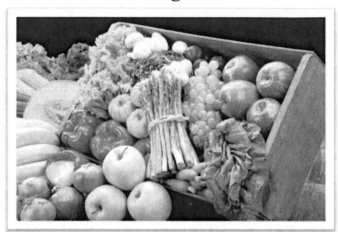

Tomatoes: Heirloom, Romano, organic-have lutein that has amazing anticancer properties.

Cruciferous vegetables: Broccoli, Cauliflower, Brussel sprouts, have amazing anti-cancer properties. They can negatively affect the thyroid unless they are lightly cooked.

Dark green leafy vegetables: Kale, Spinach, Collard and Beet greens all have amazing healing properties and if lightly cooked will not negatively affect the thyroid.

Root vegetables: carrots, beets, onions, radishes, potatoes (small and multicolored)

Zucchini squash: great for raw pasta and awesome for flavor and texture.

Cilantro: Great detoxing properties and good for your immune system.

Parsley: Great for detoxing and good for your immune system.

Dandelion greens: Great for your immune system.

Asparagus: great for your prostate and immune system.

Vital Fruits:
Seasonal, Organic and local are BEST!!
Organic and Frozen 2nd BEST!

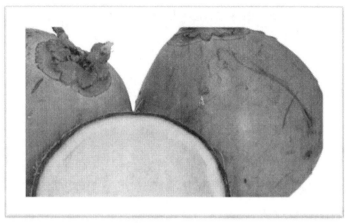

Young Thai Coconut: great for electrolytes.

Citrus: Oranges, lemons, grapefruit, limes, cumquats, etc..: Vital for your immune system.

Banana's: great for digestion and mood.

Tropical fruits: Mangos, papayas, pineapples, etc. Have great anti-inflammatory and Anti-cancerous properties.

Berries: Blue, raspberries, black, all berries: have anti-inflammatory and antioxidant effects.

Pasta Choices

Sea weed noodles: awesome for your thyroid.

Quinoa: healthy ancient grain.

Zucchini squash: great for raw pasta.

Soba Noodles: Made from Buckwheat and awesome for your immune system.

Chapter 8

One Pot/Pan Wonders

One Pot Wonders: I spend a lot of time on my boat, so I got used to making meals using only one pot. I have a steamer on top of a pot of boiling water to cook the vegetables at the same time. This saves time and energy required to cook your meals and it saves time on clean up. I'm giving you a few examples of my one pot wonder recipes. Get creative and have fun! Change the spices, add turmeric or oregano to any recipe for health and flavor.

Cacio e pepe (with or without cheese):
8oz of quinoa
1 tbs of pine nuts
1 tsp sea salt (or more if you like)
1 tsp black pepper (or more if you like it spicy)
1/3 cup organic virgin olive oil
2 handfuls of broccoli and/or asparagus
1/4 cup organic romano cheese (optional)

Boil 8 oz of quinoa pasta in a pot of filtered water until al dente. While the pasta is cooking, place the broccoli and/or asparagus in the steamer. Keep checking the veggies so they don't overcook, quinoa takes a bit more time to cook than wheat pasta.

When the pasta and veggies are done cooking, drain the pasta (don't rinse the pasta) place it back in the pot and add the olive oil, pine nuts, salt and pepper, and cheese. (optional)

Prepare the veggies with a light amount of olive oil salt and pepper serve on the side with the pasta. Serves 2

Spichatoe's

(a Bergman Family Favorite)

10 to 12 small organic colored potatoes

1/2 cup of coconut oil

4 cloves of fresh garlic

2 tsp sea salt

1 tbs black pepper

3 jalapeno's

1 lb of organic spinach

2 romano tomatoes (optional)

1/4 lb of raw cheese (optional)

Rinse the potatoes but leave the skins on. Place in large pot with filtered water enough to cover the potatoes. Chop the jalapenos and tomatoes wash and cut the spinach. Place all the veggies (except the garlic we want that raw) in the steamer over the potatoes. Be careful, the veggies may be done before the potatoes. When the potatoes are done drain and mash them. In the pot they cooked in add the veggies and minced raw garlic and coconut oil, and cheese (optional) and season to taste. Enjoy. Serves5-6

Spanish Rice one pot wonder

Spanish Rice: 2 cups filtered water

1 cup organic wild rice

3 Jalapeño chilies

3 cloves of garlic

2 Romano tomatoes

1/2 tsp turmeric

Sea salt

Black pepper

1 tbs coconut oil

In a medium sauce pan add water and rice. Bring to a boil then reduce heat to low. Add the diced jalapeno chilies & garlic. Simmer with the top on until the rice is nearly done then add the tomatoes and spices. Stirring every few minutes until rice is done. Add the coconut oil. Enjoy!   Serves 2 – 4 people

Sautéed Vegetable medley

Veggie one pot wonder:

Mix every vegetable you have and cook under low heat until al dente. Add salt and pepper to taste.

1/2 red onion or Maui onion diced

3 to 4 large cloves of garlic

2 zucchini's cut into ¼ inch strips

1 handful of cut broccoli flowers

1 large carrot cut into ¼ inch strips

2 tbs dried or fresh oregano

Sea salt (to taste)

Black pepper (to taste)

1/2 fennel root

4 asparagus spears

1/3 cup small green beans

1/4 cup of coconut oil

2 diced tomatoes (romano or heirloom)

Curcumin and turmeric (to taste)

Under low heat sauté the garlic and onions and carrots until the onions begin to change color. Add all the spices and veggies and continue to cook under low heat. Stir every minute to blend. Cook until al dente. Serve by itself or with pasta or potatoes. Enjoy!

Serves 3 to 4

Fast Veggie Dinner (*one pot wonder*)

8 carrots -cut in half and quarters length wise

5 zucchini -cut length wise in quarters

1 leek chopped

4 bell peppers- red, green, orange, yellow cut

1/4 length wise pieces

2 tbs organic coconut oil

1 tsp Celtic sea salt

1/4 tsp cayenne pepper

1/8 lb grated raw cheese (if dairy is ok for your body/condition)

Heat the coconut oil in a very large pan , toss in the carrots and seasonings first. Add the peppers, leeks, zucchini and cover. Stir the veggies every couple of min. Cook till tender yet firm for about 10 min. Sprinkle cheese just before serving. (great for next day lunches). Serves 3 – 4 people

Fast One Pot Wonder Soup

3 Chopped peppers (green, red, orange)

1/2 red onion (chopped)

4 big cloves of garlic

1 tbs. coconut oil

2 jalapeño peppers (optional)

1 box of organic fire roasted or basil tomato soup

2 packages of free range organic turkey meat

balls (if animal products are approved for you)
Sauté the veggies in the oil for 4 minutes. Pour
in the box of soup and add the turkey balls.
Heat for about 8 minutes, Just before boiling
turn down heat and simmer for about 6 min.
until the turkey balls are hot. Serves 3 – 4
people

Chapter 9: Foods for the Holidays and Healthy Pasta

Lemony Potatoes

5 lb red organic potatoes

4 lemons juiced

1/2 cup coconut oil

Sea Salt

Cayenne pepper

Wash and cut potatoes (leave the skin on) cut into ½' cubes. Spread onto cookie sheets. One layer mix 1/2 cup coconut oil, lemon juice, sea salt, cayenne pepper. Bake at 325 for about 1 hr. Turn with a spatula every 15 min. until golden brown. (Serves7 -10)

Greek Green Beans

5 lbs organic green beans

6-8 grated fresh Romano tomatoes

1/2 cup coconut oil

Green beans washed and ends cut, put in a big

pot over med heat with olive oil, tomatoes season with sea salt cayenne pepper cook until tender about an hour.
(Serves 7-10)

Garlic mashed potatoes

5 lbs organic red potatoes
1 cup coconut oil
6-10 cloves of fresh garlic
Wash and leave the skin on. Boil organic potatoes until tender then drain. Add fresh finely chopped garlic and heat garlic for just 2 min. in 1/8 cup of coconut oil. Add potatoes and mash up adding more coconut oil, sea salt and cayenne pepper to taste.
(Serves 7-10 people)

Braised Greens

2 bundles of Kale
2 bundles of collard greens

2 bundles of dandelions

3 bundles of spinach

2 lemons

1/4 cup of coconut oil

Sea Salt

Cayenne

Wash all and cross cut kale/collard to 3/4 pieces. Put in big pot over med. heat with 1/4 cup coconut oil. Season with sea salt cayenne pepper, and simmer for about 45 min. until tender, then add lemon juice.

Serves 5-8 people

Sautéed Garlic Spinach

8 bundles or 3lbs of organic spinach

1 bulb chopped garlic

1 tsp turmeric

Sea salt

Black pepper

2 tbs coconut oil

In a large pot put the coconut oil and chopped garlic over low to medium heat for 2 minutes.

Add the washed spinach, folding the oil on of the cooked spinach leaves. Add the spices while adding more of the spinach, cook until tender, and enjoy. Serves 5-8

Raw Pasta

Raw pasta can be done with seaweed noodles or any solid vegetable I like zucchini it has a great texture and accepts the flavors like pesto that you are going to add. To prepare the zucchini you will need a mandolin (not the instrument the kitchen utensil) or cut the zucchini in 1/8 to 1/16 inch strips length wise or pasta size. If you use sea weed noodles make sure you rinse them really good to soften them.

Pesto: (great for raw pasta)
2 cups of washed and dried greens (basil, lemon basil, or parsley)
1/2 cup of olive oil
3 to 4 large cloves of garlic

Sea salt (to taste)

Black pepper (to taste)

1/4 cup of pine nuts (optional)

Blend all the ingredients together in a food processor or blender and let it sit for a half hour (overnight is better) or more before using (this will add to the flavor)

Raw Pasta: Mix raw pasta choice (washed sea weed or cut zucchini) in a bowl with the pesto and enjoy.

Great for lunch or dinner (serves 2-3)

Chapter 10: Burger, Fries and Chips

Portabella Mushroom Burger

1 portabella mushroom

2 cloves of finely chopped garlic

2 slices of raw goat cheese (if dairy is ok for you)

1 sprouted grain bun or large butter lettuce leaves

1 tbs coconut oil

Layer a very thin amount of coconut oil on the bun; place the rest of the coconut oil in a medium sized pan under medium heat. Place the chopped garlic on the coconut oil and place the washed portabella mushroom on top of the garlic. Cook for about 2 minutes or until slightly tender then turn over for about 1 min. Toast the buns with the coconut oil side down for about 30 sec. Place the mushroom between the buns and enjoy. *For the breadless alternative use the butter lettuce leafs.*

French Fries

3 organic potatoes washed (but leave the skin on)

1/4 cup coconut oil

Sea salt

Cayenne pepper

Cut the potatoes into ¼ inch by ¼ inch length ways sections with a mandolin or good knife work. Heat the oil and fry until golden brown, salt and pepper to taste.

Baked Chips

3 organic potatoes or yams, washed with the skin on

1/4 cup coconut oil

Sea salt

Cayenne pepper

Cut the potatoes into 1/8 inch slices with a mandolin or good knife work, Rub the oil on a cookie sheet in a low heat over at 118 degrees for about 1 hour or until golden brown, make sure you turn them with a spatula every 10 minutes, salt and pepper to taste

Chapter 11 Awesome Deserts

Baked apples: (one apple per person)
Organic apples
Cinnamon
Wash the apples and cut the stem out by making a ½ to ¾ inch deep cut at an angle like cone, but leave the apple core in.(don't remove the core, the apple seeds have great healing properties)

Place the apples in a baking pan that has about ¼ inch of filtered water and put a generous amount of cinnamon on top of the apple in the cone shaped cut out. Bake at 350 degrees F. for about a half hour or until the apples are tender. You can eat the apples warm or save in the refrigerator for a great snack/desert.

<u>Organic chocolate desert</u>: 1 square per person (rich and satisfying, small desert)
Bakers unsweetened
Organic raw local honey

Break a square of chocolate off of the bar and dip into the honey and enjoy.

Chocolate Heaven Bars
Base:
¾ cups Dates

½ cup Coconut Oil

2 tbsp. Maple Syrup

1 tbsp. Vanilla Extract

1 ¼ cup Pecans

Combine in food processor until smooth, press mixture in your choice of pan.

Filling:
1/3 cup Coconut Oil

¾ cup Maple Syrup/Honey

¾ cup Cacao Powder

Combine in food processor until smooth, pour over base mixture, refrigerate.   Enjoy!

Coconut Cream Dream:
Meat from 2 or 3 whole young Thai coconuts

Water from 1 Thai Coconut

2 handfuls raw cashews

2 vanilla beans (scrape out and use the inner powder only)

3 tbsp. tocotrienols or rice bran soluble

2 tbsp. coconut nectar

½ cup shredded, dried coconut flakes, blended into powder

1/3 - ½ cup coconut oil

Cacao nibs.

Combine all ingredients in blender, except the cacao nibs.

Pour the blended thick cream into a bowl, sprinkle with cacao nibs.

Parfait Variation:

Pour the blended cream over a bowl of your favorite fresh seasonal chopped fruit. Enjoy!

Great fruit ice cream:

2 frozen bananas run through the masticating juicer (Champion) or in a blender add chocolate chips or fresh berries and a teaspoon

of raw cacao powder.

Healthy Tapioca:
1/4 cup of Chia seeds
1 cup of organic almond milk
3 drops of organic vanilla extract
Cinnamon (serves 2-3)

Mix the chia seeds almond milk and vanilla and place in the refrigerator in small serving cups, for 1/2 hour, the seeds will absorb 4 times their volume of the almond milk. Then sprinkle with
the cinnamon and serve. Experiment with more or less seed to get the consistency you like.

Melissa's Kettle Corn
1/2 cup organic popcorn
1/4 cup coconut oil
1/4 cup organic cane sugar
Sea Salt

Place oil and 3 kernels of corn in a large pot under medium heat. Once the kernels pop the oil is a good temperature, quickly pour the rest of the corn in the pot along with sugar. Put the lid on immediately shake the pot over the heat constantly until the popping slows down. Remove from heat add salt to taste and enjoy!

Chapter 12 Sample meals

Break fast:
#1 Egg/s with 1 tbs organic virgin coconut oil fresh clove of chopped garlic season with sea salt and cayenne pepper and sliced melted raw goat cheese

#2 Fresh fruit with berries, melon, citrus, apples (all fruit needs to be organic if you eat the peal) fruit by itself or with yogurt or granola and/or oatmeal

#3 Fresh cooked steel cut oatmeal with dried fruit, honey, cinnamon, sea salt

#4 <u>Coconut smoothie</u> – 1 Thai coconut, 1 frozen banana, 2 tbs raw cacao, 1 tbs maca root, 2 tbs spirulina powder.

Lunch:

#1. Fruit and Braised Greens with lemony potatoes

#2. Fresh Green Greek salad with grilled small wild fish

#3. Spring mixed greens with organic rice and grilled vegetables
#4. Spanish (one pot wonder chapter 8) rice, with sautéed spinach

Dinner:
#1.Braised Greens, lemony potatoes, grilled animal (optional, buffalo, grass fed beef, small wild fish, legumes,) Steamed veggies (broccoli, green beans, carrots) with raw goat cheese (if dairy is recommended), Desert: Fresh fruit by itself or with coconut ice cream.

#2.Greek green beans with garlic mashed potatoes. Desert: Fresh fruit by itself or with coconut ice cream

#3. Spichato's (one pot wonder Chapter 8)
sautéed spinach. Desert: healthy tapioca
(chapter 11)

#4. Portabella burger and sweet potato chips
(chapter 10) Desert: baked apple (chapter 11)

Chapter 13 Using Food as Medicine

Cherries- *Arthritis & Muscle pain*
Compounds in cherries called anthocyanins (the same phytonutrients that give cherries their rich ruby hue) are powerful antioxidants, block inflammation, and inhibit pain enzymes.

Ginger-*Migraines, arthritis, sore muscles*
This spicy root is a traditional stomach soother, easing seasickness, nausea, migraines, arthritis pain, and muscle aches. Use fresh or powdered ginger when you cook, or nibble on a piece or two of crystallized ginger candy daily.

Cranberry Juice- *Ulcers*
Ulcers are the result of a pathogen called H. pylori, which attacks the protective lining of the stomach or small intestine. Cranberry juice has the ability to block H. pylori from adhering to the stomach lining.

Salmon, Herring, Sardines-*Achy back, Neck, Joints*
Eating fish low in mercury and high in omega-3 fatty acids-relieve back pain.

Turmeric -*Achy joints, colitis (inflammation of the colon)*
Relieves pain and speeds up digestion. Turmeric also acts as an anti-inflammatory.

Yogurt-*Irritable Bowel Syndrome (IBS)-*
Yogurt will help to replace the healthy bacteria and may reduce pain, inflammation, and bloating.

Coffee-*Headaches, constipation-*can reduce prostate and endometrial cancers. *Journal Cancer Epidemiology Biomarkers and Prevention* found that women who drank more than four cups of coffee a day had a 25 percent lower risk of endometrial cancer. Coffee contains many biologically active compounds, including caffeine and phenolic acids that have potent antioxidant activity and can affect glucose metabolism and sex hormone levels. Because of these biological activities, coffee may be associated with a reduced risk of prostate cancer

Mint-*IBS, Headaches, Pain, muscle spasms, insect bites or stings.*
Chewing on peppermint can freshen your breath. A drop of peppermint essential oil

rubbed into the center of a bite or sting can bring quick, longlasting relief.

Brewing mint tea- *For pain.*
Pour boiling water over peppermint leaves and steep until the tea is as strong as you like. Add wintergreen leaves for an extra pain-fighting boost; squeeze of lemon will help you extract as many pain-reducing chemicals as possible from the plants.

Hot Peppers-*Arthritis*
An ingredient in hot peppers called capsaicin does the trick by stimulating nerve endings and depleting a chemical that relays pain signals.

Cayenne Pepper- topical relief is most effective for arthritis, eating hot peppers also yields pain-fighting benefits. Mix cayenne with hand cream for a great heat generating and pain reliever, be careful to not get any in a cut or on sensitive area's it can burn.

Turmeric *–Heartburn*
Take two or three turmeric capsules (1/2 to 1 g) before a meal.

Thyme- has expectorant and antibacterial properties. It helps to protect the respiratory system and effective disinfectant and excellent treatment for bacterial acne.

Rosemary- *Headaches*
Brew rosemary as a tea. Use 1 teaspoon of rosemary per cup of hot water. Cover, and steep for 10 minutes. Strain, and sip a cup three times a day headaches

Cloves- *Toothache*
Rub a drop of essential oil of clove directly on an aching tooth or just wiggle a whole clove, pointed end down, next to the tooth.

Natural Antibiotics

Cloves (Clove Oil)
digestive disorders, diarrhea, athlete's foot and other fungal infections, oral antiseptic

Colloidal Silver
Hippocrates was one of the first to describe its antimicrobial properties in 400 B.C. successfully combat otherwise antibiotic-resistant bacteria

Echinacea
microbial infections, inflammation, it is often effective against both bacterial and viral attacks.

Garlic
used throughout history as an effective antibiotic antifungal, anti-parasitic, anti-protozoan, and antiviral

Oregon Grape Root

a great treatment for sore throats, disorders of the stomach, intestines, urinary organs, eczema, herpes, psoriasis, acne, and pimples

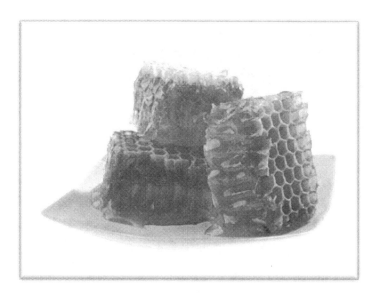

Raw Honey

Raw honey, which has not been pasteurized or filtered, can be especially useful for medicinal, antibiotic purposes, to sooth a sore throat and ease a cough, treat minor cuts, scrapes and burns by applying directly to the affected area, and as a healing mask for blemished prone skin.

Mullein

Help to reduce upper respiratory infection symptoms, such as fatigue, sore throat, cough and headache.

Myrrh

Myrrh has been used by natural

healers for hundreds of years. It's antiseptic, antibiotic and antiviral properties. It can be taken internally and used externally as a gargle or wash for wounds.

Sage
Among the Ancients and throughout the Middle Ages, healing ailments of the mouth, teeth, blood, joints, liver, urine, head, sinuses, throat, lungs, and stomach.

Powerful way to Knockout a Cold or Flu
First Sign of a cold:

1. Stop eating solid foods (try the super soup recipe with extra garlic and turmeric)
2. Start Drinking Lots of water and teas
3. Lots of dark green veggie juice (spinach, apples, carrots, celery)
4. Build your Fever (hot baths, Special Tea [recipe below]
5. Exercise as soon as you feel up to it
6. Take 50,000 IUof vitamin D-3 for 5 days
7. Take 2000 mg of vitamin C daily for at least 5 days

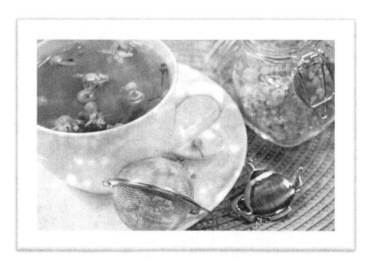

Super Tea for cold's and flu's

1 oz sliced fresh ginger
1 broken-up cinnamon stick
1 teaspoon coriander seeds
3 whole cloves
1 lemon slice
1 pint water

Simmer for 15 minutes and straining. Then drink a hot cupful every 2 hours.

Heat Generating Tea:

Lemon (squeeze 1-2)
Ginger (small piece about the size of your
   thumb)
Cayenne pepper (Dash to taste)
Peppermint (handful of leaves or fresh
   oregano)

Heat up and steep for a few min. make it hot but not too hot do drink quickly

How to Heal Foot Fungi

Toe/foot/nail fungus several methods:
- Clean the blood (vegan, lots of water, colonic)
- Eliminate processed foods, sugars and breads
- Cut the nails close
- Apply aloe vera 2 times a day

50/50 vinegar water soak:
- 1 part Vinegar to 2 parts water
- Soaks= 45 min for 2 weeks change aloe/ vinegar every 4-5 days

More methods for healthy feet:
- Tea tree oil 2 times a day
- Oregano oil
- Vicks vapor rub
- Use baking soda has foot powder for dryness

Antibiotic Alternatives

Beetroot – A beetroot is rich in folic acid, very low in calories and is said to contain loads of antioxidants

Flaxseed- Flaxseed is very inexpensive and can be added to breads, oatmeal or even as a topping for cereal. Due to the high levels of fiber in flaxseed, it has been known to have laxative properties and helps to detoxify the digestive system by ensuring proper waste elimination.

Garlic- Garlic is an essential detoxifier due to its antiviral, antiseptic and antibiotic properties. Garlic can be eaten a number of ways; however, you must know that garlic needs to be sliced, cooked or chewed before its healing abilities become activated.

Nettle- Nettle is an herbaceous perennial flowering plant that helps to cleanse the urinary system and help prevent any recurring urinary issues. Nettle is known as a mild diuretic, is high in vitamins and minerals, including iron and aids in blood purification. Often, nettle can be found in tea form.

Dandelion- Dandelion is used as a cleanser for the gallbladder and liver. It is also a very rich source of vitamins and minerals, including vitamins A, D, C, and B, plus iron, silicon, magnesium, zinc and manganese. Dandelion reduces inflammation and infection and can even aid movement in your bowels because it helps the gallbladder produce bile.

Final Chapter and Notes

When it comes to diet advice, everywhere you look there are different theories. When looking at diets, you need to consider how sustainable they are. By "sustainable" I mean what type of impact this type of diet would have on the eco-system of our planet. I recommend diets that are plant based, whole, unprocessed, organic and seasonal foods. Below are some of the diets that are out there and why I like or dislike them:

Paleo Diet (caveman diet)- People on the Paleo diet eat meats, nuts, seeds, fruit, and they avoid grains, refined sugars, salt, potatoes and legumes. The good parts of this diet is eliminating refined salts and sugars. The challenge I have with this is the planet wouldn't be able to sustain the amount of animals needed if we all ate this diet.

Vegan diet – Vegans only plants. No dairy, no fish, no animals. The good part of this diet is that it's great for the planet and great for humans. The challenge is that most cultures have an addiction to meat and many societies have both dairy and animals as part of their culture. According to the Price-Pottenger Foundation there are no vegan cultures on the planet. All cultures have some type of animal, animal product or insects on their menu.

Vegetarian (Ovo, lacto) – Vegetarians eat plants. Ovo-vegetarians eat plants and eggs. Lacto-vegetarians eat plants and dairy. Ovo-Lacto-vegetarians eat plants eggs, and dairy. The good part of all 3 types of vegetarian diets is that they are very sustainable and good for the planet. The only challenge with the vegetarian type of diet is that some people can gain weight from too many grains. This is probably the best choice of diet for our planet and overall health.

Whole Food Diet - Weston A. Price was a dentist who traveled the world to observe native cultures in the 1930's. He found that even though each culture had different diets they shared certain traits. Each culture ate *local whole, unprocessed, organic, seasonal, foods*. In the cultures that he observed there were few to no degenerative disease. He found cultures that ate modern refined foods had the most degenerative diseases. He studied Eskimo's, Polynesians, Swiss, African's, virtually every climate and type of traditional culture.

The Great Starch/Grain Debate

Dr. John McDougall and Dr. Joel Fuhrman are brilliant Doctors who have differing ideas on nutrition. I like parts of both of their theories. Where Dr. McDougal is a proponent of starches, Dr. Fuhrman is a proponent of a vegan lifestyle. They do agree on a few points:

- Get the poisons out of the diet
- Eat whole foods
- Eat healthy starches
- Eat a plant-based diet

Natural Cancer Therapies Differ in Diet suggestions- Each of the methods below are effective for different types of cancer. I picked these because they have such differing views on the types of diet for healing. By bringing this up I just want you to appreciate that there may be more than one "right diet". For health and disease reversal find what works for you.

The following is a few examples of diet recommendations for healing:

Gerson Therapy – uses a vegan diet.

William Kelly Method – uses raw liver shakes

Budwig Method – uses cottage cheese and flax oil

All of the diets have a few things in common

I have given you just a few recipes to start a healthy diet and restore your health. This is not a complete list of the benefits that healthy eating can give you, but it's just a guide to get you started. With all of the different and conflicting ideas on what is a healthy diet, just go to back to the basics. The factors of the best diets are:

- Eliminate Genetically Modified Foods (GMO's)
- Eliminate processed foods
- Eliminate refined grains
- Must have a plant based organic diet
- Any animal products must be from healthy animals and less than 10% of your calorie intake
- Have a clean water source

In addition to a healthy diet, there are 4 more vital aspects to health:

1. **Nerve Supply**-Your body rebuilds itself

every 90 days by having mental impulses from the brain flow down to the tissue cells. If this vital information flow is choked off, Dis-ease is the result.

2. **Exercise-**is vital to rid your body of waste products and reverse the dis-ease processes.

3. **Rest** - is when your body actually rebuilds itself. Under normal sleep you have between 6-8 periods of R.E.M. state of sleep. During R.E.M sleep is the deep sleep when rebuilding occurs.

4. **Prayer and Meditation** -increases cell production, maintains the connection with your source.

To change the world you have to begin with changing yourself. Choosing what you eat can change our planet and have a global impact.

Eating the right, healthy foods will leave you feeling healthy and energized. Know that what you eat becomes you!

Let's make a difference! Change your health thereby change the world!

Dr. John Bergman

NOTES

NOTES

NOTES

NOTES

NOTES

NOTES

NOTES

NOTES

NOTES

Special Thanks and appreciation for their input in this book:

Melissa Douglass

Dr. John Dewitt D.C.

Nikki Jeannine Stewart is a Certified Natural Health Professional and a Certified Digestive Health Specialist. She has designed a comprehensive program to help you develop your own personalized health and wellness lifestyle that is simple, easy and fun to follow. www.FrequencyofUltimateHealth.com

My Sons:

Michael Bergman

Danny Bergman

And my Mom, Bette Bergman

For more information go to our web site at:

www.owners-guide.com

And check out other books by Dr. John Bergman

All available on Amazon in Paperback or Kindle version:

"How to Reverse Arthritis Naturally" a #1 Best Seller

"How to Correct High Blood Pressure Without Medications" a Best Seller

"How to Recover From Fibromyalgia, Real Solutions for a Real Problem"

"How to Save Lives Through Marketing"

I am also available for one-on-one skype/phone consultations.

Go to

skypepackage.com

for packages and pricing.

CPSIA information can be obtained at www.ICGtesting.com
Printed in the USA
LVOW07s2331260314

379058LV00029B/1576/P